Natural Homemade Skincare Recipes:

Amazing recipes for shiny skin

Judy Cinta

TABLE OF CONTENT

INTRODUCTION

"Unlock the secrets to radiant and healthy skin with ' Natural Homemade Skincare Recipes.' This comprehensive guide is your gateway to a world of pure, nurturing ingredients that harness the power of nature for a revitalized complexion. Delve into a collection of carefully curated recipes that blend science with simplicity, allowing you to craft your very own skincare concoctions right in the comfort of your home.

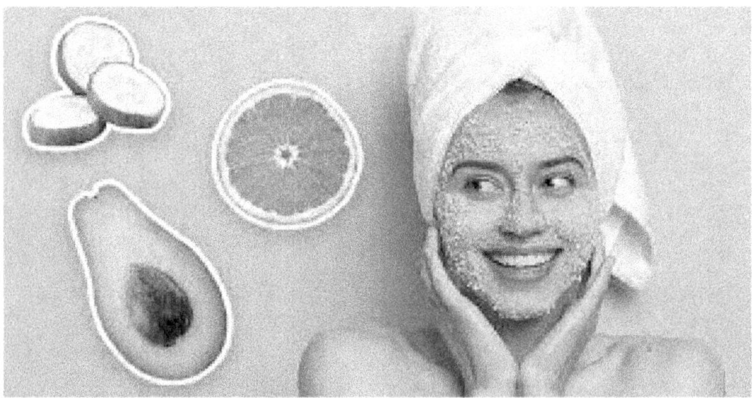

Each chapter unveils a selection of easy-to-follow recipes, from cleansers that gently purify to masks that invigorate and moisturizers that rejuvenate. Dive into the transformative properties of ingredients like honey, oatmeal, avocado, and more as you discover the wonders of crafting personalized skincare solutions that cater to your unique needs. Whether you're seeking an escape from commercial products laden with chemicals or a deeper connection with your skin's natural beauty, this book is your companion on the journey to self-care and radiance. Embrace the art of mindful skincare and unveil a vibrant, glowing you through the harmonious blend of nature and nurture."

Chapter 1

Cleansers

Cleansers in natural homemade skincare recipes are essential products used to cleanse the skin and remove dirt, oil, and impurities. Typically made from natural ingredients like honey, yogurt, oils, or aloe vera, these cleansers are gentler on the skin and avoid harsh chemicals found in commercial alternatives. They aim to promote a balanced complexion while avoiding potential irritants, making them a popular choice for those seeking a holistic skincare approach.

1. Honey and Lemon Cleanser:

Honey and lemon serve as natural cleansers. Honey moisturizes and soothes, while lemon's citric acid gently exfoliates, promoting clear skin without harsh chemicals.

Procedure

Mix 1 tablespoon of raw honey with a few drops of lemon juice. Massage onto damp skin, then leave for 5-10 minutes before you rinse off with warm water.

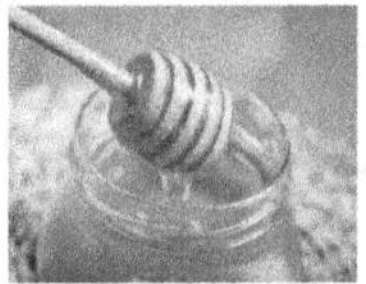

Honey

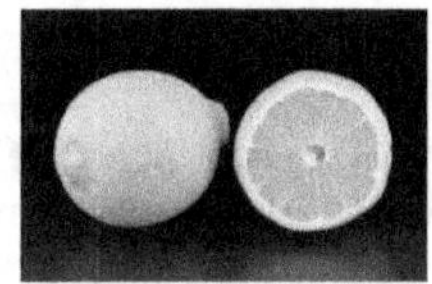

lemon

2. Milk and Honey Cleanser:

A Milk and Honey Cleanser is a natural skincare product blending milk's nutrients and honey's antibacterial properties for gentle cleansing and hydration.

- Mix 1 tablespoon of milk (any type) with 1 teaspoon of honey. Apply to your face, gently massage, leave on the face for about 1 - 2 minutes and gently rinse with lukewarm water.

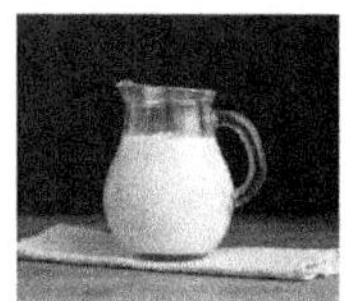

Milk

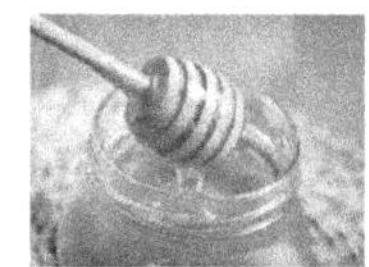

Honey

3. **Yogurt and Cucumber Cleanser**:

A yogurt and cucumber cleanser is a homemade skincare solution that uses these ingredients to gently cleanse, soothe, and hydrate the skin.

- Blend 2 tablespoons of plain yogurt with a few slices of cucumber. Apply to your face, massage, and rinse.

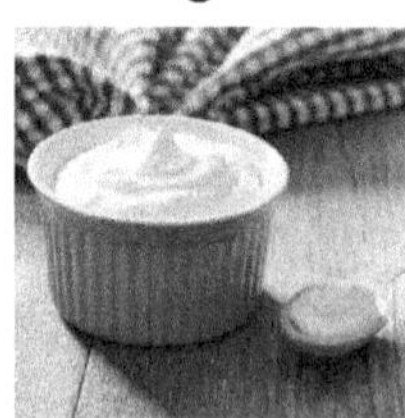

Yoghurt

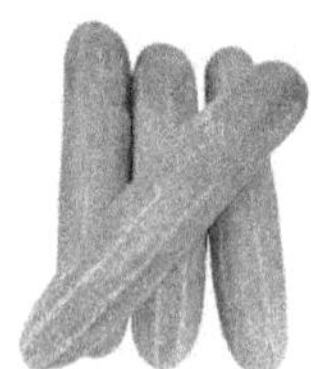

Cucumber

Chapter 2
Exfoliator

Exfoliators in natural skincare recipes are gentle products that remove dead skin cells, promoting smoother skin. Common ingredients include sugar, oats, or coffee grounds, offering a cost-effective and chemical-free option for rejuvenation.

1. Brown Sugar and Olive Oil Scrub:

Brown sugar and olive oil scrub is a natural exfoliator that blends coarse brown sugar with moisturizing olive oil, effectively removing dead skin cells while hydrating the skin for a smoother texture.

Procedures

- Mix 2 tablespoons of brown sugar with 1 tablespoon of olive oil. Gently scrub onto your skin, then rinse.

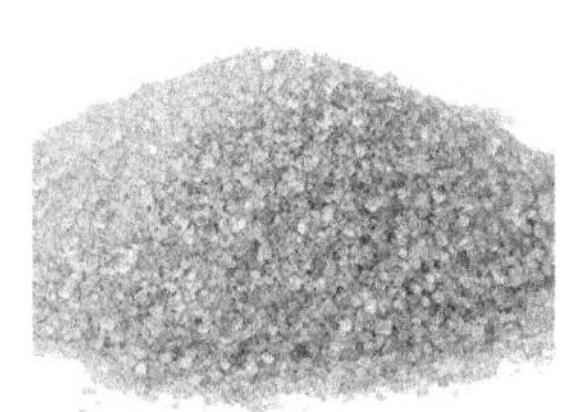 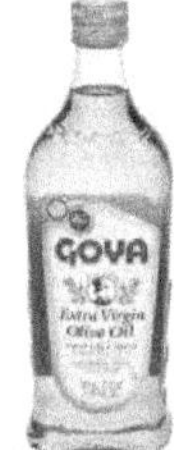

Brown sugar   **olive oil**

2. Coffee Grounds Scrub:

Coffee grounds scrub exfoliators use coarse coffee particles to remove dead skin, enhance circulation, and provide a natural, invigorating exfoliation.

Procedures

- Mix used coffee grounds with a bit of water or coconut oil to create a scrub. Gently massage onto your skin, then rinse.

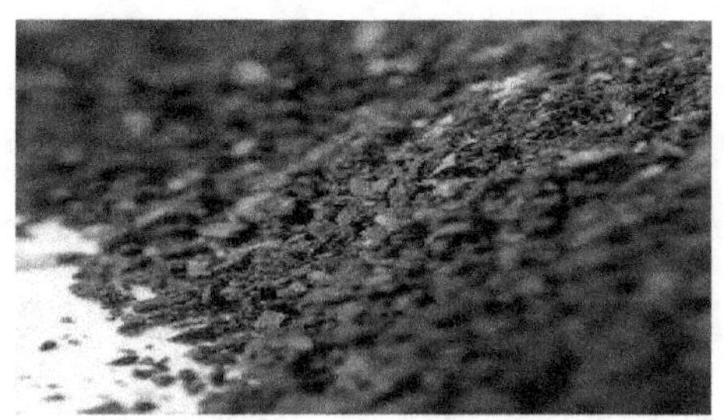

3. Oatmeal and Banana Scrub:

Oatmeal and banana scrub exfoliators combine oats' gentle exfoliation with banana's nutrients, leaving skin softer, hydrated, and refreshed.

Procedures

- Blend 1/2 ripe banana with 2 tablespoons of oatmeal. Apply the mixture to your skin, massage, and rinse.

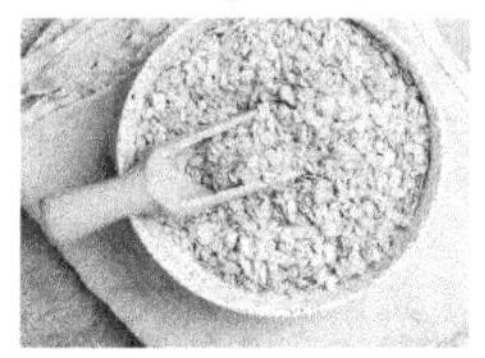

oatmeal

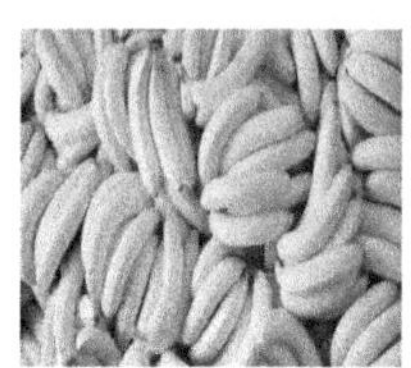

Banana

Chapter 3

Masks

Masks in homemade skincare recipes are topical treatments made from natural ingredients. Applied to the face, they can address various skin concerns like hydration, exfoliation, or calming, enhancing overall complexion and health.

1. Turmeric and Yogurt Mask:

Turmeric and yogurt mask is a natural skincare remedy. Turmeric's anti-inflammatory properties combined with yogurt's soothing effect promote clear and radiant skin.

Plain, unsweetened yogurt is best for turmeric and yogurt masks.

Procedures

- Mix 1 teaspoon of turmeric with 2 tablespoons of yogurt. Apply, leave on for 10-15 minutes, and rinse.

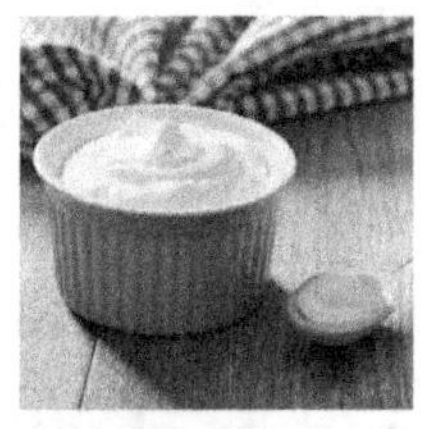

Yoghurt

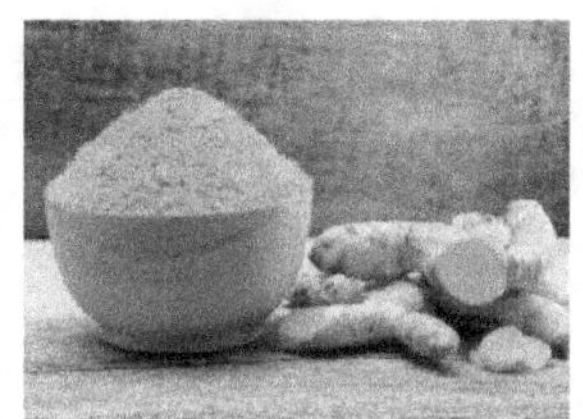

Turmeric

2. Aloe Vera and Cucumber Mask:

An Aloe Vera and Cucumber mask is a soothing homemade skincare remedy that combines their hydrating properties to refresh and moisturize the skin.

Procedure

- Blend aloe vera gel with cucumber juice. Apply, leave on for 15-20 minutes, and rinse.

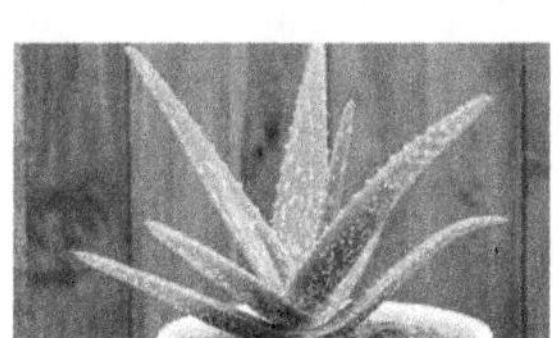

Aloe vera

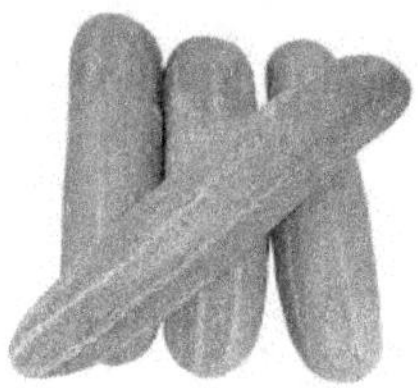

Cucumber

3. Egg White and Lemon Mask:

An Egg White and Lemon Mask is a natural skincare remedy, combining egg whites and lemon juice to tighten pores and brighten skin tone.

Procedure

Beat an egg white with a few drops of lemon juice. Apply, let dry, and rinse off.

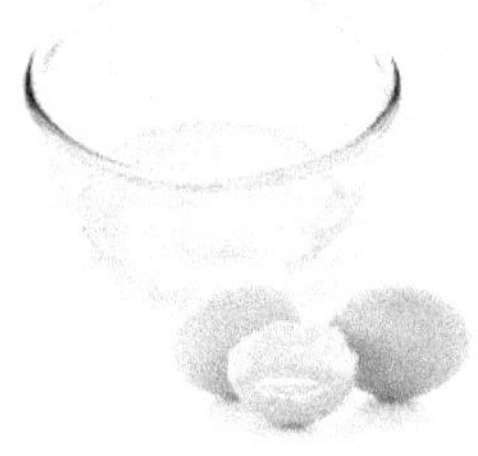

Egg white

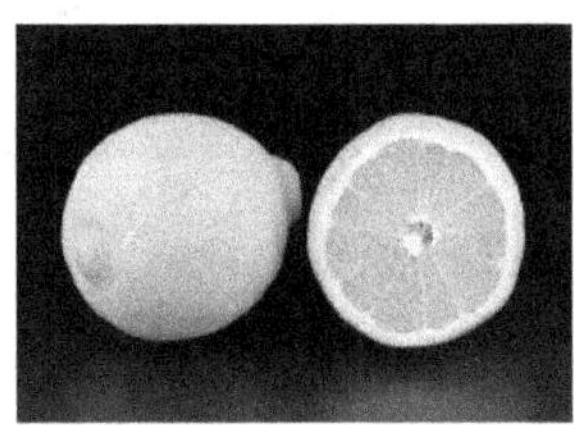

Lemon

Chapter 4
Toners

Toners in natural skincare recipes are liquids applied after cleansing. They balance skin pH, tighten pores, and prep for moisturizers. Common homemade toners include rose water, green tea, and apple cider vinegar.

1. Apple Cider Vinegar Toner:

Apple cider vinegar toner is a natural solution made by diluting ACV with water. It balances skin pH, reduces acne, and clarifies complexion.

Procedure

Dilute 1 part apple cider vinegar with 3 parts water. Apply to skin with a cotton pad after cleansing.

Note;

"3 parts water" means that you would mix three times the amount of water compared to the amount of apple cider vinegar. For example, if you use 1 tablespoon of apple cider vinegar, you would mix it with 3 tablespoons of water. This dilution helps prevent the ACV from being too strong for your skin.

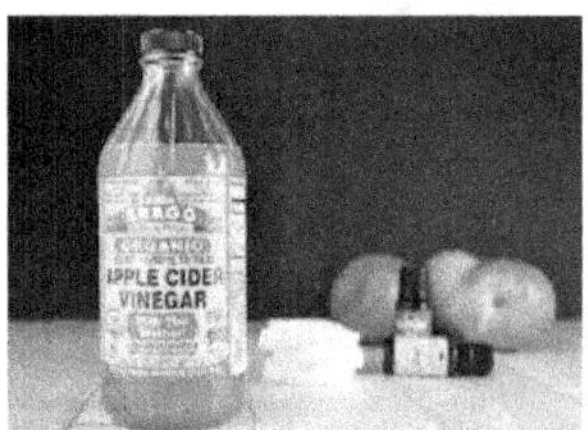

Apple Cider Vinegar Toner

2. Rose Water Toner:

Rose water toner, a natural homemade skincare staple, is derived from roses. It soothes, hydrates, and refreshes skin, offering a gentle and fragrant way to maintain skin health.

Use pure rose water as a toner to refresh and hydrate your skin.

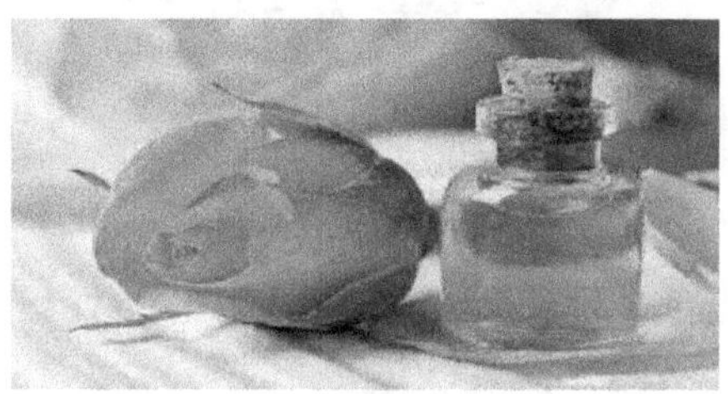

Rose water

3. Green Tea Toner:

Green tea toner is a natural DIY skincare product made from steeped green tea. It soothes, hydrates, and calms the skin.

Procedure

Brew green tea, let it cool, and use it as a toner for its antioxidants.

Leave green tea toner on your face for about 5-10 minutes before rinsing. Adjust time based on your skin's sensitivity.

Chapter 5
Moisturizers

Moisturizers in homemade skincare recipes provide hydration, nourishing the skin with natural ingredients like oils, butters, and aloe vera. They help maintain skin's moisture balance, promoting a healthier complexion.

1. Coconut Oil Moisturizer:

Coconut oil moisturizer is a simple, natural skincare recipe. It utilizes pure coconut oil to hydrate and soften skin, leaving it radiant and smooth.

Combine 1/2 cup coconut oil with 1 tsp vitamin E oil. Mix, store in a jar. Apply as needed for natural skin hydration.

- Apply a small amount of melted coconut oil to your face and body.

Leave coconut oil moisturizer on your skin for at least 30 minutes to absorb fully. You can also leave it on overnight for deeper hydration.

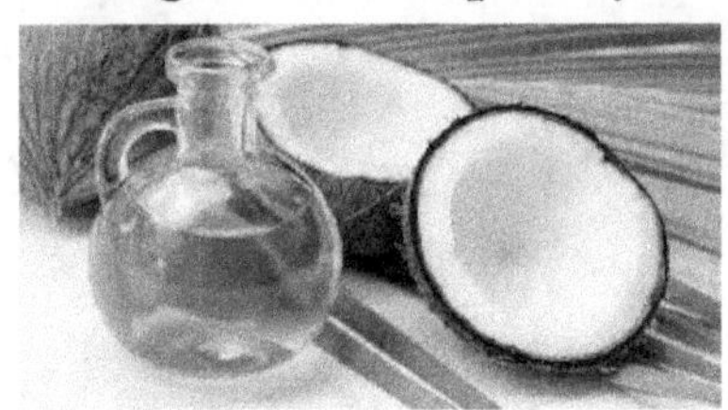

2. Shea Butter Moisturizer:

Shea butter moisturizer, a natural homemade skin care remedy, uses shea butter's rich, fatty acids to deeply hydrate, soften, and protect the skin.

To make Shea Butter Moisturizer, melt 1/2 cup of raw shea butter, blend with 1/4 cup of coconut oil, and add a few drops of essential oil. Cool, then store in a jar.

- Gently warm shea butter and apply it to dry areas for deep moisturization.

Shea butter moisturizer is typically not washed off. Apply a small amount to clean, dry skin and leave it on to absorb for the best results.

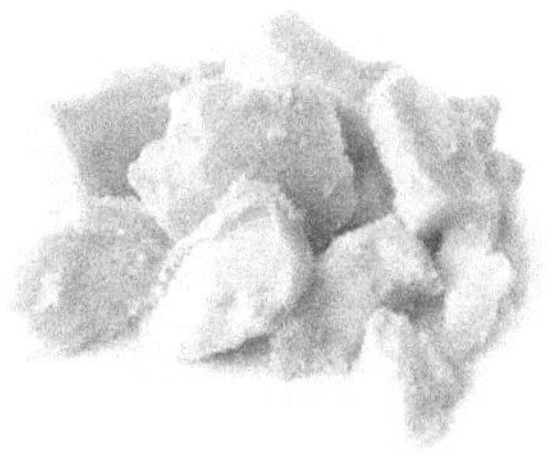

Shea butter

3. Jojoba Oil Moisturizer:

Jojoba oil moisturizer, a natural DIY skin care remedy, hydrates skin deeply due to its resemblance to skin's natural oils, promoting softness and balance.

Jojoba oil is not made at home; it's extracted from jojoba seeds through a commercial process. The seeds are cold-pressed to yield the liquid oil, which is a valuable skincare ingredient.

Apply a few drops of jojoba oil to damp skin to lock in moisture.

Jojoba oil is typically used as a leave-on product, not requiring washing off. Apply a small amount to clean skin, and it can be left on throughout the day or overnight for maximum moisturizing benefits.

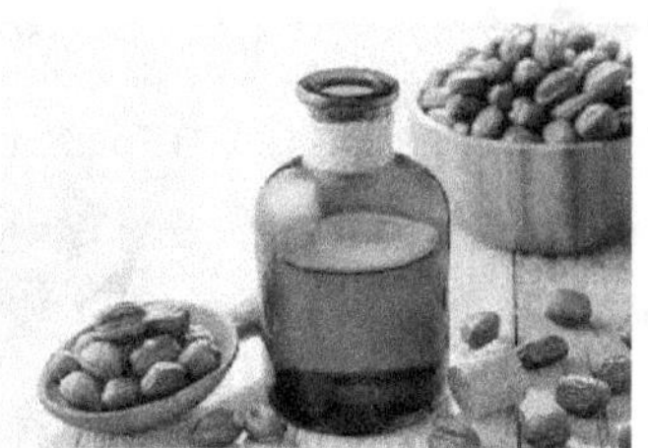

Jojoba oil

Chapter 6

Serums

Serums in natural homemade skincare recipes are concentrated, lightweight liquids infused with beneficial ingredients like oils, vitamins, and antioxidants. They target specific skin concerns, offering potent nourishment and hydration for a healthier complexion.

1.Vitamin E Serum:

Vitamin E serum in homemade skincare is a potent blend of vitamin E oil, often mixed with carrier oils, to moisturize and rejuvenate skin, providing antioxidant protection.
Mix vitamin E oil (puncture a capsule) with jojoba oil (2 tbsp) and lavender oil (5 drops). Apply nightly for nourished skin.

Leave the vitamin E serum on your skin overnight for best results. It can be used as an overnight treatment without rinsing.

2. Hyaluronic Acid Serum:

Hyaluronic Acid Serum enhances homemade skincare with deep hydration, promoting a plump and youthful complexion, often used in DIY recipes.

Mix distilled water, hyaluronic acid powder, and optional glycerin. Heat, stir, and store in a dark glass bottle for DIY serum..
Apply hyaluronic acid serum to clean skin, then leave it on. Don't wash it off; it's designed to be left on for maximum hydration.

Chapter 7
Lip Care

1.Brown Sugar Lip Scrub:

A DIY skin care staple, it exfoliates and moisturizes lips using brown sugar, honey, and coconut oil.

Mix brown sugar and honey (or coconut oil) in a bowl, then apply gently to lips, massaging for exfoliation, and rinse.

You can leave Brown Sugar Lip Scrub on your lips for about 1-2 minutes before gently washing it off. This gives the sugar granules enough time to exfoliate your lips, and then you can rinse to reveal smoother, softer lips.

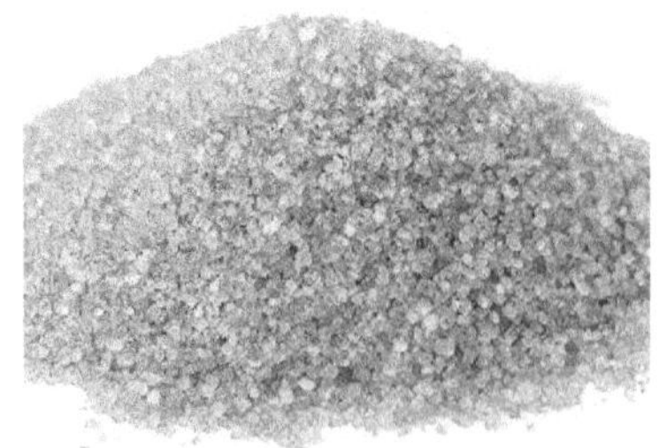

2. Coconut Oil Lip Balm:

Coconut oil lip balm is a natural, hydrating lip care product enriched with coconut oil to moisturize, soothe, and protect dry or chapped lips.

- Melt coconut oil with a bit of beeswax for a natural lip balm.

Coconut oil lip balm is typically not meant to be washed off. It's used to moisturize and protect your lips. You can apply it as often as needed throughout the day to keep your lips hydrated. If you find it feels too heavy or you want to remove it, you can wipe it off gently with a soft cloth or tissue. Otherwise, it's safe to leave on your lips for extended periods.

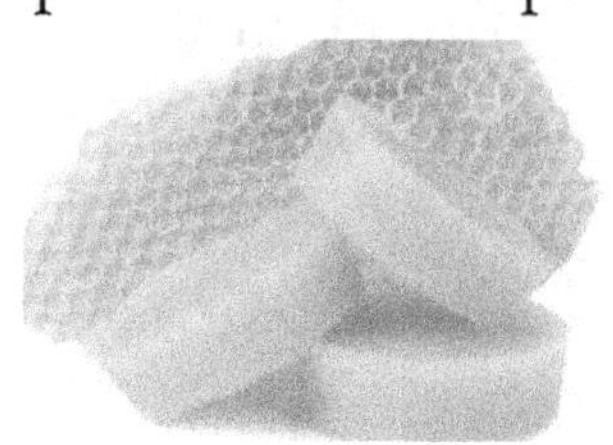

Beeswax

Chapter 8
Under-EyeTreatments

Under-eye treatments are skincare products designed to address concerns like dark circles, puffiness, and wrinkles. They often contain ingredients like hyaluronic acid, peptides, and antioxidants to rejuvenate the delicate under-eye area.

1.Cucumbers and Potato Eye Mask:
Cucumbers and potatoes are used in homemade skincare masks to reduce puffiness and dark circles. Their natural ingredients soothe and rejuvenate the under-eye area.

- Blend cucumber and potato, apply the mixture under your eyes, leave it on for 10-15 minutes, and rinse.

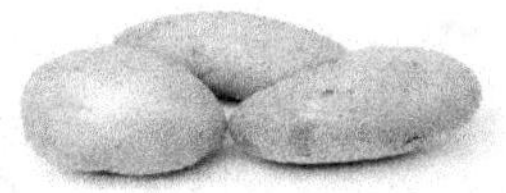

potatoes

2. Green Tea Bags:

Green tea bags are used in homemade skincare for their antioxidant properties. They can reduce inflammation, soothe skin, and help treat issues like dark circles when applied topically.

- To make green tea bags, steep green tea leaves in hot water for 2-3 minutes, then allow them to cool before placing them on your eyes..

To use green tea bags for your eyelids, steep them in hot water, then cool and apply to closed eyelids for about 10-15 minutes before gently removing.

Remember that consistency is key when using homemade skincare products. Everyone's skin is different, so pay attention to how your skin responds and adjust the recipes as needed. If you have specific skin concerns or sensitivities, consider consulting a dermatologist before trying new skincare recipes.